LUNG CANCER DECODED:

A Comprehensive guide to understanding the causes, diagnosis symptoms & treatments of lung cancer

By

TONY R. WALKER

Copyright © by Tony R. Walker, 2023. All rights reserved.

TABLE OF CONTENTS

INTRODUCTION

"Lung Cancer Decoded" is a comprehensive guide that aims to shed light on every aspect of this prevalent disease by exploring its causes, symptoms, diagnosis, treatment options, dietary considerations, and coping strategies. This book will equip patients and their loved ones with the knowledge and tools necessary to navigate this challenging journey. Lung cancer, one of the most common and formidable forms of cancer, affects millions of lives worldwide. Its impact reaches far beyond the individual diagnosed, touching the hearts and minds of families, friends, and communities. However, knowledge is power, and arming ourselves with a deep understanding of this disease enables us to confront it with resilience and hope. Within the pages of this book, we will journey through the intricate web of lung cancer, unraveling its origins and exploring the diverse factors that contribute to its development. We will explore the signs and symptoms that may serve as early warning signs, empowering individuals to seek timely medical attention.

Furthermore, we will delve into the various diagnostic techniques utilized by medical professionals, ensuring that no stone is left unturned in the pursuit of accurate and timely detection.

Treatment options are an essential aspect of any discussion surrounding cancer, and lung cancer is no exception. In "Breathe," we will navigate the diverse array of treatments available, from surgery and radiation therapy to targeted therapies and immunotherapy. We will explore the latest advancements in medical science, providing a comprehensive overview of potential treatment paths, their benefits, and their limitations. Recognizing that healing encompasses more than medical intervention alone, this book also delves into dietary considerations that can complement the treatment process. We will explore the role of nutrition in supporting the body's healing mechanisms and discuss strategies for maintaining a balanced, nourishing diet during and after treatment.

 Finally, This book acknowledges the emotional and psychological toll that lung cancer can have on individuals and their loved ones. We will explore coping strategies and support systems, empowering readers to cultivate resilience and find solace amidst the challenges they may encounter. I invite you to join me on this enlightening and empowering journey through the intricacies of lung cancer. Together, let us unveil the mysteries, empower lives, and foster a compassionate community that stands united in the face of adversity.

"Lung Cancer Decoded" is a testament to the human spirit's indomitable strength, providing a beacon of hope and knowledge for all those touched by lung cancer.

CHAPTER 1

WHAT IS LUNG CANCER?

Lung cancer Is a type of cancer that affects the lungs. The two spongy organs in the chest that are responsible for breathing in oxygen and exhaling carbon dioxide are the lungs. It starts in the lungs and has the potential to move to other body organs.

Additionally, cancer can spread to the lungs from other body organs.

Anyone can be affected by lung cancer. Lung cancer typically affects older adults, with an average age of diagnosis being around 70 years old.

What leads to lung cancer?

Lung cancer is caused by breathing in hazardous and poisonous substances.

Here are the main causes of lung cancer.
Smoking

Smoking is the main source of lung cancer. Individuals who smoke have the most serious gamble of cellular breakdown in the lungs. Lung cancer can likewise happen in individuals who have never smoked. The risk of having lung cancer increases with the period of time and number of cigarettes you've smoked. If you quit smoking, even in the wake of smoking for a long time, you can fundamentally diminish your possibilities, creating a cellular breakdown in the lungs.

It causes around 90% of cellular breakdown in lung cases. Tobacco smoke contains numerous synthetic compounds that are known to cause cellular breakdown in the lungs. Assuming you actually smoke, stopping smoking is the absolute smartest option for your lung well-being.

Smokers are not by any means the only ones impacted by tobacco smoke. Your risk of developing lung cancer has decreased if you stopped smoking, but it has not completely subsided. Non-smokers can additionally be impacted. Taking in handed-down cigarette smoke endangers you with cellular breakdown in the lungs or different diseases.

Exposure to dangerous chemicals and radioactive gasses

The second biggest cause of lung cancer is naturally occurring radioactive gasses like radon.

Such gasses cause lung damage equivalent to that of smoking.

On the other hand, there is a risk of lung cancer from exposure to dangerous chemicals. If you are not properly covered, working with chemicals such as nickel, arsenic, uranium, and even dust and vapors can be extremely harmful.

Genetic components

One's risk of lung cancer may also be influenced by genetic factors. You may be more likely to get lung cancer if there is a family history of the illness.

A small number of lung cancers are linked to genes. You may already know that genes are pieces of DNA that carry the instructions your body needs to work. Genes control how your cells grow, divide, and die. Oncogenes are a type of gene that helps cells grow and divide. Tumor suppressor genes stop cells from dividing or make them die off when you don't need them anymore.

Changes called mutations in these genes allow cells to divide and divide until they form tumors. That's how cancer starts.

Some gene mutations make it harder for your body to get rid of cancer-causing chemicals. Others prevent damaged DNA from repairing itself.

Most gene changes that raise lung cancer risk happen during a person's lifetime. Rarely someone inherits these mutations from their parents. Genes are more likely to cause some types of lung cancer than others.

Types of lung cancer
There are two main types of lung cancer.
1. Non-small cell lung cancer (NSCLC)
About 80% to 85% of lung cancers are NSCLC. The main subtypes of NSCLC are adenocarcinoma, squamous cell carcinoma, and large cell carcinoma.

These subtypes, which start from different types of lung cells, are grouped together as NSCLC because their treatment and prognosis are often similar.

Adenocarcinoma: Adenocarcinomas start in the cells that would normally secrete substances such as mucus. This type of lung cancer occurs mainly in people who smoke or used to smoke, but it is also the most common type of lung cancer seen in people who don't smoke. It is more common in women than in men, and it is more likely to occur in younger people than other types of lung cancer. Adenocarcinoma is usually found in the outer parts of the lung and is more likely to be found before it has spread. People with a type of adenocarcinoma called adenocarcinoma in situ tend to have a better outlook than those with other types of lung cancer.

Squamous cell carcinoma: Squamous cells are flat cells that line the lining of the lungs' airways. Squamous cell carcinomas begin in these cells. They are typically located in the middle of the lungs, close to a major airway, and are frequently associated with a history of smoking.

Large cell carcinoma: This type of lung cancer can develop anywhere in the lung. It can be more difficult to treat because of its tendency to grow and spread swiftly. Large cell neuroendocrine carcinoma (LCNEC) is a fast-growing subtype of big cell carcinoma that has many characteristics with small cell lung cancer.

Additional subtypes: Certain other subtypes of non-small cell lung cancer, like sarcomatoid carcinoma and adenosquamous carcinoma, are far less common.

2. Small Cell Lung Cancer (SCLC)

SCLC accounts for 10% to 15% of all lung cancer cases. It's also referred to as oat cell cancer. SCLC is characterized by rapidly proliferating tiny cells that form tumors in the central areas of the lungs. Unlike non-small cell lung cancer (NSCLC), surgical intervention is less prevalent in this type of lung cancer because it is frequently detected after it has progressed to other organs. Instead, a mix of radiation therapy and chemotherapy is usually used as part of the treatment. In some circumstances, immunotherapy may also be employed.

CHAPTER 2

SYMPTOMS OF LUNG CANCER

Early detection of lung cancer greatly increases the likelihood of a favorable outcome. It is essential to comprehend the signs of this illness in order to diagnose it early and take appropriate action.

The following are the most typical signs of lung cancer.

1. Persistent Cough: For several weeks or even months, a persistent cough is one of the most typical signs of lung cancer. Over time, this cough may get worse, and some people may get a persistent cough that discharges phlegm that is rust- or blood-colored. In the event that your cough becomes more severe or prolonged, you need to see a doctor.

2. Shortness of Breath: Dyspnea, or shortness of breath, is a symptom of lung cancer. It could develop as a result of a tumor constricting or obstructing the airways, making breathing difficult. This symptom frequently gets worse with physical activity or as the illness worsens.

3. Chest aches and pains: Chest aches and pains that are prolonged or get worse over time may be a sign of lung cancer.

The lungs, the chest wall, or the tissue surrounding the lungs could be the source of the pain. Chest discomfort associated with lung cancer can be mild, aching, or severe, and deep breathing, coughing, or laughing can exacerbate the pain.

4. Unexplained Weight Loss: Patients with lung cancer frequently have inadvertent weight loss. This weight loss, which can happen quickly, is frequently accompanied by weakness, exhaustion, and muscle atrophy. You should speak with a healthcare provider if you lose a lot of weight for no apparent reason.

5. Fatigue and Weakness: Lung cancer may be the cause of persistent fatigue and weakness.
Cancer cells experience numerous energy-draining processes. Furthermore, weakness and exhaustion may be the outcome of the body's immunological reaction to the malignancy.

6. Hoarseness and Vocal Changes: Vocal cord function-related nerves and airways can be affected by lung cancer, which can result in hoarseness or vocal changes. Lung cancer might sometimes cause voice alterations that are persistent or inexplicable.

7. Recurrent Infections: People with lung cancer are more prone to infections like pneumonia or bronchitis because lung cancer can impair immunity.

It is important to look into respiratory infections that are recurring or frequent.

8. Wheezing: Patients with lung cancer may experience wheezing, a high-pitched whistling sound made during breathing. It may be brought on by inflammation or a tumor, causing the airways to constrict.

9. Clubbing of the Fingernails: The expansion and rounding of the nails and fingertips are the hallmarks of the clubbing condition. It has been linked to a number of lung conditions, including lung cancer. Clubbing can be a late-stage symptom of lung cancer and is brought on by an inadequate oxygen supply to the fingers.

10. Bone Pain: Bones are one area of the body where advanced lung cancer may spread. For example, bone metastases in the spine, hips, and ribs can result in localized discomfort that is frequently intense and chronic.

CHAPTER 3

HOW LUNG CANCER IS DIAGNOSED

How lung cancer is diagnosed
There are several ways to diagnose lung cancer.
Which are :
1. Imaging procedures to detect lung cancer
Imaging tests produce images of your interior organs using radioactive materials, sound waves, magnetic fields, and X-rays. Before or after a lung cancer diagnosis, imaging studies may be performed for a variety of reasons, including:

1. To examine regions that seem worrisome or could be cancerous
2. To determine the potential spread of the malignancy
3. To assess if the treatment is effective.
4. To search for any indications that the cancer may recur following treatment.

X-ray of the chest: Often, your doctor may start by doing a chest x-ray to check for any abnormalities in the lungs. Your doctor might prescribe more testing if they find anything unusual.

CT (Computerized Tomography) scan: A CT scan creates fine-grained cross-sectional images of your body using X-rays. Unlike a traditional X-ray which only takes one or two images, a CT scanner collects numerous images, which are then combined by a computer to display a portion of the body being examined.

Lung cancers are more visible on a CT scan than on a standard chest x-ray. It can also help identify enlarged lymph nodes that may contain cancer and display the location, size, and form of any lung tumors. Additionally, this test can be used to search for masses that may be related to the spread of lung cancer in the liver, brain, adrenal glands, and other organs.

CT-guided needle biopsy: When taking a tissue sample for cancer testing from a suspected cancerous location deep within your body, a CT scan may be utilized to guide the biopsy needle into the area. A scan using magnetic resonance imaging (MRI) MRI scans provides fine-grained images of the body's soft tissues, just like CT scans do. However, an MRI scan substitutes radio waves and powerful magnets for X-rays. The most common use of MRI scans is to check for potential lung cancer metastases to the brain or spinal cord.

Positron emission tomography (PET) scan:
FDG, a mildly radioactive sugar, is administered into the bloodstream prior to a PET scan, and it primarily gathers in cancer cells.

PET/CT scan: Using a specialized device that can perform both simultaneously, a PET scan and a CT scan are frequently combined. This enables the physician to contrast regions of increased radioactivity on the PET scan with a more comprehensive image on the CT scan. Patients with lung cancer are most frequently scanned with this sort of PET scan.

CT and PET scans can be helpful. If a medical professional believes the cancer may have spread but is unsure of its location. They may demonstrate the spread of malignancy to the adrenal glands, liver, bones, or other organs. They are less effective when examining the brain or spinal cord. Their significance in determining whether treatment is effective is unknown, although they are useful in identifying lung cancer. PET/CT scans are not typically advised by doctors for normal patient follow-up following lung cancer treatment.

Bone scan:A tiny quantity of low-level radioactive material is put into the bloodstream for a bone scan, and it primarily gathers in aberrant bone regions.

If cancer has gone to the bones, it may be visible using a bone scan.

However, PET scans can typically detect bone metastases of cancer. Therefore, this test is rarely necessary.

2. Carrying out tests to diagnose lung cancer

Although a person's symptoms and test results may strongly indicate that they have lung cancer, lung cells in a lab are used to make the official diagnosis. The cells can be extracted from lung secretions, which are the mucus that comes out of the lungs when you cough, from a suspicious location using a needle or during surgery, or from any combination of these procedures. The circumstance will determine the test or tests to use.

Cytology of Sputum: Mucus that is coughed out from the lungs is called sputum. The purpose of the lab examination is to detect cancerous cells in a sample of sputum. It is advisable to obtain samples early in the morning, three days in a row. Squamous cell lung tumors, for example, are more likely to be detected with this test than other types of lung cancer that originate in the main airways. For the detection of other forms of lung cancer, it might not be as useful. Even in the event that no cancer cells are discovered in the sputum, additional testing will be conducted if your doctor suspects lung cancer.

Thoracentesis: Doctors can remove part of the fluid that has accumulated around the lungs to determine whether the fluid is the result of cancer spreading to the pleura, the lining that lines the lungs. Other illnesses like heart failure or an infection could potentially be the source of the accumulation.

A hollow needle is placed between the ribs during a thoracentesis procedure to drain the fluid after the skin has been numbed. In the lab, the fluid is examined for cancerous cells. Different fluid tests can occasionally be helpful in distinguishing between a malignant (cancerous) pleural effusion and a non-cancerous one. Following a diagnosis of malignant pleural effusion that is impairing breathing, a second thoracentesis may be performed to remove additional fluid, potentially improving breathing.

Needle biopsy: A hollow needle is frequently used by doctors to take a little sample from a questionable area. The fact that needle biopsies don't need a surgical incision is one of their advantages.

The disadvantage is that they only remove a tiny quantity of tissue, and in certain situations, the tissue may not be sufficient to diagnose the disease and to conduct additional tests on the cancer cells that would aid in the selection of anticancer medications by medical professionals.

Biopsy using fine needle aspiration (FNA): A syringe with a very thin, hollow needle is used by the physician to extract tiny tissue fragments and cells to examine for cancer in the lymph nodes that connect the lungs, a FNA biopsy may be performed.

Transtracheal FNA, also known as transbronchial FNA: It is performed by inserting the needle through the wall of the trachea or bronchi. In certain cases, an endoscopic esophageal ultrasonography involves a FNA biopsy performed by inserting a needle through the esophagus wall.

Core biopsy: A bigger needle is employed to remove one or more tiny cores of tissue. Because core biopsies are larger than FNA samples, they are frequently selected.

Needle biopsy in the thoracic cavity: If the suspected tumor is in the lungs' outer layers, the biopsy needle can be inserted through the skin on the chest wall. Local anesthesia may be used to numb the area where the needle will be put first. The doctor then guides the needle into the location while using fluoroscopy or a CT scan to examine the lungs. This technique may result in air leaking out of the lung at the biopsy site and into the gap between the lung and the chest wall. This is known as a pneumothorax. It can cause a portion of the lung to collapse and, in certain cases, difficulty breathing. If the air leak is minor, it usually resolves on its own. Large air leaks are addressed by inserting a chest tube (a short tube into the chest space) that sucks out the air for a day or two before healing on its own.

Bronchoscopy: Bronchoscopy can aid the doctor in the detection of tumors or obstructions in the bigger airways of the lungs, which are frequently biopsied during the operation.

If lung cancer is discovered, it is often necessary to determine whether it has progressed to the lymph nodes in the space between the lungs or to other surrounding locations. This can have an impact on a person's treatment options. Several sorts of tests can be performed to detect the spread of cancer.

Endobronchial ultrasonography: If biopsies are needed in the space between the lungs, endobronchial ultrasonography can be utilized to see the lymph nodes and other structures.

Endoscopic esophageal ultrasonography:Endoscopic esophageal ultrasonography is a type of endoscopic esophageal ultrasound.
Endoscopic esophageal ultrasonography examines the esophagus, revealing surrounding lymph nodes that may contain lung cancer cells.
Mediastinoscopy and mediastinotomy are both medical procedures.

These procedures can be used to acquire a closer look at samples from the structures in the mediastinum. The primary distinction between the two is the placement and size of the incision. A mediastinoscopy is a procedure that involves inserting a lighted tube beneath the sternum (breast bone) and in front of the windpipe to examine and collect tissue samples from the lymph nodes along the windpipe and the major bronchial tube locations. If some lymph nodes cannot be accessed via mediastinoscopy, the surgeon may perform a mediastinotomy to directly extract the biopsy sample. A slightly bigger incision between the left second and third ribs, near the breast bone, is required for this treatment.

Thoracoscopy: Thoracoscopy can be used to determine whether cancer has spread to the gaps between the lungs and the chest wall, as well as the linings of these spaces. It can also be used to sample tumors on the lungs' outer surfaces, as well as surrounding lymph nodes and fluid, and to determine whether a tumor is spreading to nearby tissues or organs. This treatment is rarely performed only to diagnose lung cancer unless other diagnostics, such as needle biopsies, are unable to get sufficient samples for the diagnosis. Thoracoscopy can also be used to remove a portion of a lung in some early-stage lung malignancies.

This procedure is described in Surgery for Non-Small Cell Lung Cancer as video-assisted thoracic surgery (VATS).

Lung Function Examinations

 Lung function tests, also called Lung Function Tests (PFTs), are frequently performed after lung cancer is detected to determine how well your lungs are functioning.

 This is especially crucial if surgery is a treatment option for the cancer.

 Surgery to treat lung cancer may require the removal of part or all of a lung, so it's important to know how well your lungs perform beforehand. Some persons with low lung function, like those with smoking-related lung disease, do not have enough undamaged lungs to sustain even partial lung removal. These tests can give the surgeon an idea of whether surgery is a good option and, if so, how much lung can safely be removed.

There are different types of PFTs, but they all basically have you breathe in and out through a tube that is connected to a machine that measures airflow. Sometimes, PFTs are coupled with a test called an arterial blood gas. In this test, blood is removed from an artery, unlike other blood tests in which blood is removed from the vein, so the amount of oxygen and carbon dioxide can be measured.

Lab tests of biopsy

Samples that have been collected during biopsies or other tests are sent to a pathology lab. A pathologist, a doctor who uses lab tests to diagnose diseases such as cancer, will look at the samples and may do other special tests to help better classify the cancer.

Cancers from other organs also can spread to the lungs. It's very important to find out where the cancer started because treatment is different depending on the type of cancer.

CHAPTER 4

HOW LUNG CANCER IS TREATED

Treating lung cancer

Lung cancer treatment necessitates a multifaceted approach that takes into account a variety of aspects, including the type and stage of the cancer, the patient's overall health, and customized considerations. Lung cancer treatments include surgery, radiation therapy, chemotherapy, targeted Therapy, immunotherapy, and palliative care. Depending on the features of the tumor and the patient's health, these modalities can be utilized alone or in combination. Early detection, correct diagnosis, and the selection of the most appropriate treatment strategy are all required for successful lung cancer treatment.

The treatment goal changes according to the stages of the cancer.

In early-stage lung cancer, the emphasis is frequently on curative purposes, with the goal of entirely removing the tumor and preventing its return.

The emphasis on advanced-stage lung cancer switches to extending survival, treating symptoms, and increasing the patient's quality of life.

Significant advances in lung cancer treatment have been made throughout the years, resulting in higher outcomes and overall survival rates.
Surgical techniques have improved, allowing for less intrusive treatments with less postoperative discomfort and quicker recovery times. Radiation therapy and chemotherapy have also advanced, allowing for more specific cancer cell targeting while reducing damage to healthy tissues.

Moreover, the emergence of targeted therapies and immunotherapies has revolutionized the treatment landscape for lung cancer. These innovative approaches aim to specifically target genetic mutations or activate the patient's immune system to recognize and destroy cancer cells.

Targeted therapies have shown remarkable success in treating certain types of lung cancer with specific genetic alterations, while immunotherapies have demonstrated significant efficacy in advanced-stage lung cancer, leading to prolonged survival and improved quality of life for some patients. Despite these advancements, challenges remain in effectively treating lung cancer, especially in advanced cases where the disease has spread.
The development of resistance to treatments, limited treatment options for certain subtypes of lung cancer, and the need for more personalized and tailored

therapies are areas of ongoing research and exploration.

Here are the ways of treating lung cancer
1. Surgery:

Surgical intervention is often the preferred treatment option for early-stage lung cancer. If the tumor is localized and has not spread to nearby lymph nodes or distant organs, surgical removal of the tumor and surrounding tissues can be curative.

The decision to perform surgery for lung cancer is based on several factors, including the stage of the disease, the location and size of the tumor, the patient's overall health, and individualized considerations. Surgery is generally considered the primary treatment option for patients with early-stage lung cancer, where the tumor is confined to the lungs and has not spread to nearby lymph nodes or distant organs. It is also an option for selected cases of locally advanced lung cancer.

Below are the surgical techniques
Lobectomy: Lobectomy involves the removal of an entire lobe of the lung containing the tumor. It is the most common surgical procedure for lung cancer. The remaining healthy lung tissue compensates for the loss of the lobe, and normal lung function is often preserved.

Pneumonectomy: Pneumonectomy is the removal of an entire lung.

It is typically reserved for cases where the tumor involves the main bronchus or when the cancer affects a large portion of the lung.

After a pneumonectomy, the remaining lung expands to accommodate the lost lung's function.

Segmentectomy/Wedge Resection: Segmentectomy involves the removal of a segment of the lung containing the tumor, while wedge resection involves the removal of a small, wedge-shaped portion of the lung. These procedures are considered when the tumor is small and peripheral, and lung function preservation is a priority.

Minimally Invasive Techniques: Minimally invasive surgeries, such as video-assisted thoracoscopic surgery (VATS) and robotic-assisted surgery, have gained popularity in recent years.

These techniques involve smaller incisions, resulting in reduced pain, shorter hospital stays, and faster recovery times compared to traditional open surgery. However, it is crucial to note that surgery alone may not be sufficient for advanced-stage lung cancer, where the disease has spread beyond the lungs.

In such cases, surgery may be combined with other treatment modalities, such as chemotherapy, radiation therapy, targeted Therapy, or immunotherapy, to achieve the best possible outcomes.

2. Radiation Therapy

High-energy radiation is used in this therapeutic approach to kill cancer cells or shrink tumors. Radiation therapy can be used as a primary treatment for early-stage lung cancer or as a follow-up therapy after surgery to eradicate any leftover cancer cells.

3. Chemotherapy

Chemotherapy uses chemicals to kill cancer cells. It is routinely utilized in situations of both early-stage and advanced lung cancer. Chemotherapy can be used to decrease tumors before surgery, to kill leftover cancer cells after surgery, or as the primary treatment for advanced-stage lung cancer.

4. Targeted Therapy

Targeted medicines target specific molecular abnormalities in cancer cells.

These medicines function by interfering with cancer cell development and spread while causing minimal damage to healthy cells. Targeted medicines are highly effective in treating NSCLC with specific genetic alterations.

5. Immunotherapy

Immunotherapy uses the immune system of the body to fight cancer cells. It activates the immune system, causing it to recognize and destroy cancer cells.

Immune checkpoint inhibitors, a kind of immunotherapy, have proven to be extremely effective in treating advanced-stage NSCLC and have dramatically increased survival rates.

While advances in lung cancer treatment have improved outcomes and survival rates dramatically, the concept of a universal "cure" for lung cancer remains complicated. The likelihood of a cure is determined by a number of factors, including the stage of cancer at the time of diagnosis, the precise type and genetic profile of the tumor, and the overall health of the individual patient.

For early-stage lung cancer, where the tumor is confined to the lungs and has not spread extensively, surgical resection can often result in a complete cure. However, once lung cancer progresses to advanced stages and spreads to other organs, achieving a complete cure becomes challenging.

That said, significant progress has been made in recent years. Targeted therapies and immunotherapies have revolutionized lung cancer treatment and substantially prolonged survival for some patients. Ongoing research and clinical trials continue to explore innovative treatment strategies, with the hope of achieving long-term remission or even a cure for a broader range of lung cancer patients.

CHAPTER 5

LIVING WITH LUNG CANCER

Lung cancer can be a difficult and complex journey, both physically and emotionally. Lung cancer is a serious disease that necessitates careful management and care. It is very important to focus on a healthy lifestyle and food choices that promote overall well-being. **Dietary considerations (What should I eat and what should I avoid)**

What should I eat?

There is no particular diet that can cure or even treat lung cancer. However, you can give yourself an advantage during treatment and beyond by eating smart foods that will nourish your body and help you maintain your strength. Eating a well-balanced diet may help with therapy tolerance, strength maintenance during treatment, and recovery time.

But keep in mind that the right diet isn't a one-size-fits-all prescription. Foods that are effective for your type and stage of lung cancer may not be effective for everyone else with the disease. Every lung cancer is unique. The optimum diet for you is determined by your personal objectives. If you're preparing to have lung cancer surgery, your dietary demands will be different than while you're recovering from Therapy.

Still, there are general rules you can follow while making dietary decisions.
The guidelines are as follows:

Consume enough protein: Protein is required by your body for cell and tissue repair. Protein is the building block of your immune system and is required for your organs to function properly.

Consuming fruits and vegetables: A plant-based diet is required. Colorful fruits and vegetables provide powerful antioxidants and phytonutrients to your diet, which can aid in cell protection. It makes little difference whether you eat your fruits and veggies raw or cooked; the key is diversity.

Choose whole grains: Carbohydrates are required to keep your energy levels stable. Get your carbs from whole grains rather than refined grains.
Good alternatives include:
1.\Wholegrain bread
2. Oatmeal
3. Whole-wheat pasta
4. Rice

Include good fats: Not all fats are created equal. Omega-3 fatty acids and other healthy fats aid your brain and neurological system by reducing inflammation.

These options include:
 1. Avocados
 2. Nuts
 3. Seeds
 4. Olive oil

What kinds of food should I avoid?

 As a lung cancer patient, it's critical to focus on eating a good, balanced diet to improve your overall health and treatment outcomes. While no specific foods directly cause or cure lung cancer, the following is some general advice for foods to limit or avoid:

1. Processed Meats: Consumption of processed meats such as hot dogs, sausages, bacon, and deli meats should be limited or avoided. These items frequently include excessive quantities of preservatives and additives that may be harmful to your health.

2. Sugary meals and Beverages: Reduce your consumption of sugary meals and beverages, such as sodas, sports drinks, sweetened juices, candies, and pastries. High sugar consumption can lead to weight gain and have a bad impact on your overall health.

3. Red and Processed Meats: Although there is no solid evidence linking red meat consumption to lung cancer, it is generally recommended that you restrict your intake.
 Choose lean protein sources such as poultry, fish, beans, and lentils.

 4. High-Fat Foods: Limit your intake of high-fat foods, especially those high in dangerous saturated and trans-fats. Fried foods, processed snacks, full-fat dairy products, and fatty cuts of meat are examples. Instead, choose healthier fats like avocados, nuts, seeds, and olive oil.

 5. Sodium and Salt: Avoid foods high in sodium and added salts, such as processed and packaged foods, which can cause fluid retention and high blood pressure. Instead, season your foods with herbs, spices, and other flavorings.

 6. Alcohol: Limit or prevent alcohol use because it may interfere with some medications and have a bad impact on your overall health. If you prefer to drink, do it in moderation and in accordance with health authorities' recommendations. Individual dietary demands and limits may differ depending on factors such as overall health, treatment plans, and personal preferences.

 It is best to speak with a licensed dietician or healthcare expert who can provide specialized advice geared to your specific situation.
 Concentrate on feeding your body a well-balanced diet rich in fruits, vegetables, whole grains, lean proteins, and healthy fats. Throughout your lung cancer journey, stay hydrated, eat thoughtfully, and pay attention to your body's requirements.

Coping with lung cancer emotionally

 Coping with lung cancer emotionally can be difficult, as a cancer diagnosis generally brings up a wide range of emotions.
 Here are some coping strategies for the emotional side of living with lung cancer:

1. Seek assistance: Seek emotional assistance from loved ones, friends, and support groups. Sharing your feelings, concerns, and fears with those who understand or have experienced similar situations can bring comfort and affirmation. Consider attending in-person or online support groups where you may connect with other lung cancer patients and survivors.

2. Communicate Openly: It is important to communicate well with your healthcare staff. Be upfront and honest about your feelings, concerns, and inquiries.

They can help you negotiate the emotional effect of your diagnosis by providing information, direction, and support.

3. Educate Yourself: Understanding your situation might make you feel less fearful and anxious. Discover more about lung cancer, treatment choices, and potential side effects. Understanding what to expect will help you make educated decisions and engage actively in your care.

4. Practice Self-Care: Make self-care activities that improve emotional well-being a priority. Engage in enjoyable activities such as hobbies, reading, listening to music, or spending time in nature.
Take breaks when needed, use relaxing techniques such as deep breathing or meditation, and make sure you get enough rest and sleep.

5. Express Yourself: Find healthy outlets for your feelings. Consider journaling, art therapy, or expressive writing to help you process your emotions. Engaging in creative pursuits can serve as a source of self-expression and emotional release.

6. Consider Counseling or Therapy: Professional counseling or Therapy can help you manage the emotional problems of living with lung cancer.

A therapist can provide a safe and supportive environment in which you can explore your feelings, develop coping techniques, and negotiate the complicated emotions connected with your diagnosis.

 7. Have a happy Mindset: While it is normal to feel a variety of emotions, aim to have a happy mindset. Surround yourself with positive influences, cultivate appreciation, and celebrate tiny accomplishments along the way.

 Remember that dealing with lung cancer is a personal journey, and it's normal to have good and terrible days. Allow yourself time to grieve, reflect, and adjust to the changes that come with the diagnosis. Reach out for help when you need it, and keep in mind that you are not alone on this road.

Conclusion

In conclusion, this book has explored the comprehensive landscape of lung cancer, covering its diagnosis, symptoms, treatments, and dietary considerations. Throughout its pages, we have gained valuable insights into the complex nature of this devastating disease and the various approaches to managing and combating it.

Lung cancer, as we have come to understand, is a formidable adversary characterized by its insidious development and often late-stage diagnosis. The symptoms can be subtle or easily mistaken for other ailments, making early detection crucial for improving outcomes.

By familiarizing ourselves with the warning signs discussed in this book, such as persistent coughing, chest pain, or unexplained weight loss, we can empower ourselves and others to seek timely medical attention. Diagnosis plays an indispensable role in formulating an effective treatment plan. From conventional methods like imaging tests and biopsies to emerging technologies, such as liquid biopsies and molecular profiling, advancements in diagnostic techniques are enhancing our ability to identify lung cancer subtypes and tailor therapies accordingly.

By understanding the diagnostic process outlined in this book, individuals can actively participate in their own healthcare journeys. The treatment landscape for lung cancer is continually evolving, offering hope to patients and their loved ones. Surgical interventions, radiation therapy, chemotherapy, targeted therapies, and immunotherapies have all demonstrated successes in different scenarios.

In this book, we have shed light on the potential benefits, risks, and considerations associated with each approach, enabling patients and their healthcare teams to make informed decisions. Importantly, this book has emphasized the role of diet in lung cancer management. While nutrition alone cannot cure the disease, adopting a healthy and balanced diet can provide support during treatment and contribute to overall well-being.

By incorporating evidence-based dietary recommendations, such as consuming a variety of fruits and vegetables, maintaining a healthy weight, and limiting processed foods, individuals can optimize their nutritional status and potentially enhance their body's resilience.

This book has aimed to empower readers with knowledge and understanding of lung cancer, its diagnosis, symptoms, treatments, and dietary considerations.

By cultivating awareness, encouraging early detection, facilitating informed decision-making, and promoting holistic well-being, we hope to contribute to the ongoing fight against lung cancer. Together, with continued research, education, and support, we can strive for improved outcomes and a brighter future for those affected by this challenging disease.